The Fat Trainer® Diet and Exercise Plan

L Duhigg

When you are tired of how you feel. You will make the changes.

Find an exercise you love and throw your heart and soul into it

If I can do it – you can too!

HEALTHY weight loss takes time and commitment.

How committed are you to a lifestyle change?

The best piece of advice I can give you ?

Big changes start with small steps

ISBN-10: 1505352975
ISBN-13: 978-1505352979

DEDICATION

To Vickie – The real reason the sun rises each and every morning

To all of my clients both past and present - there isn't a day that goes by
that I don't learn as much from you as you learn from me

To Jessica – "Not all Trainers start out thin" are words I have lived by since
the day you spoke them

To Angela and Judy – Thanks for believing in me

It's time to get this party started!

This book contains the opinions and ideas of the author. It is intended to provide helpful and informative material on the subjects addressed in this book and is sold with the understanding that the author and publisher are not engaged in rendering any kind of personal or professional services in this book. The author and publisher disclaim all responsibility for any liability, loss or risk, personal or otherwise, that is incurred as a consequence, directly or indirectly, of the use and application of any of the contents of this book. This book does NOT replace the advice or direction of health care providers or qualified medical or mental health professionals.

CONTENTS

ACKNOWLEDGMENTS

For each and every person that stumbles and falls while on the path to a healthier and fitter version of themselves.

If it were easy – everyone would be doing it.

1 THE FAT TRAINER ®

I was lucky enough to grow up during a time when kids didn't worry much about body image or concern themselves with calories or eating for wellness.

My diet was relatively healthy because fast food and processed food was not yet a staple. Most meals were prepared using whole ingredients and eating out was reserved for special occasions.

I did suffer from a sugar addiction that could rival the most addicted personality out there. I loved sugar. It was as important to me as breathing but my mother and father really did not allow us to consume many sweets.

My desire for sugar was so strong that I remember eating teaspoons of sugar straight from the sugar bowl. During the summer my daily snack consisted of a piece of white bread drenched in maple syrup.

As a kid and young adult my activity level offset my occasional poor eating habits. As I aged I became less active and after a major injury that required a long recovery, my meals began to consist of drive-thru and processed sugar. I packed on weight and blamed my pants being too tight on irregular clothing purchases.

Eventually I grew comfortable with my larger size. My new larger shape gave me strength and power. I was able to move large heavy things with little effort. I was also absolved from the continual pushy advances from guys that thought they were every woman's personal gift.

I remember the first time I heard the term "Morbidly Obese". I was visiting a doctor for a lower back issue. The doctor told me if I lost weight and stopped wearing tight pants, my back pain would likely disappear. "Effects of Morbid Obesity" was my official diagnosis. I watched as he scribbled the words across the page. I was young enough that the words didn't faze me. I shrugged it off and continued living my life with back pain.

As I began to age, I began to feel more and more pain. My lower back, neck, shoulders, hips, knees and feet were in a continual state of discomfort.

Moving from one room to another became a chore and I would need to rest once I made the ten foot trip. I would need to lean on a desk or dresser for support while catching my breath. I thought I was catching a cold or had the flu.

Denial is a beautiful thing. Or is it.

My life change one day in March of 2007. I was going to take a friend to the airport during a blizzard when I was involved in a head on collision.

I entered the intersection and gasped as I heard the roar of an engine. I saw a green Tahoe flying toward me. I knew it was icy and I had little chance of stopping but still tried to step on my break. The other drivers' engine roared and he tried to power through the inevitable. His vehicle went into a slide and slammed into mine. I don't recall much at that point but I do recall the sound of metal bending around metal and I recall a noise louder than anything I have ever heard radiating throughout my entire body clear down to my soul and then nothing but a blasting ringing through my ears.

My knees hit the steering wheel column and my neck rocked back and forth. As I sat taking inventory of my body, the aches and pains started creeping in but reality was still disconnected from the event.

My vehicle was also a Tahoe that became nothing more than a large paperweight upon impact of these two giant beasts.

I remember two people coming to the driver's door. A man and a woman. They were talking but I couldn't hear them over the ringing in my ears. As I tried to roll the driver's side window down they kept talking. I pointed to my ears and told them I couldn't hear them and motioned to my ear. I remember being frustrated with the driver's window and assumed the motor wasn't working. It wasn't until later that I learned that the window had been shattered when my head bounced off of it.

I remember the woman telling the man 'She's in shock. They better get here soon." But I didn't comprehend at the time who or what they were talking about.

I decided to get out of the vehicle and see how bad the damage was. As I stepped on to the ice and felt the sting of the blowing wind and snow I felt the world start to spin. I walked to the front of my Tahoe. I remember being upset at the sight of the crumpled hood and began to feel faint. I knew I needed to sit down or I would pass out so I got back in the vehicle.

Not long after, I heard sirens and vaguely recall being swarmed by paramedics. One moment I was in my vehicle and the next I was laying in the back of an ambulance being whisked to a nearby hospital.

"Do you have car insurance miss?" A man's voice demanded a response. I remember hearing the words and not understanding the meaning. He kept repeating his question and I remember the female paramedic telling him to sit down and be quiet. She asked me to look at her. I couldn't. I saw nothing but fog. Her voice becoming an echo. I wanted to close my eyes and as I started to, a jolt of urgency flooded through my body. I knew if I closed my eyes that would be the end of me.

People write about near death experiences all of the time. White lights, peace and calm. Someone on the other side waiting for them.

This isn't that story.

As I lay in the ambulance while it made its way through the blizzard and ice covered roads I heard blasts of the siren. How easy it would be to close my eyes and finally go "home". Something I had wanted since I was a little kid. I never felt I belonged in this world and at that moment, I felt I was being given an out. If I closed my eyes, I would be done here. But…...

My family was out of town on another medical issue. They were clear across the country. My dogs and cats had no one to take care of them. The dogs were hyper protective of the house so if I died, no one would be able to get in the home to help them and it would take my family 2 days to get there.

The blasts of siren, the paramedic asking about my pain level which was accompanied the man's voice demanding my insurance information – drifted away and everything chaotic became calm and quiet. The pain disappeared and I felt warm and peaceful. I was aware of the noise and drama but I only "heard" what was in my own head.

"I have to stay here God. My pets need me. They have no one to take care of them. I can't leave them. It will take Vickie 2 days to get home and she can't really leave because of what's happening out there. She needs to be there. My pets need me and I can't leave. I just can't. I'll do anything you want. I'll be anything you want but please let me stay. You HAVE to know that it's important if I WANT to stay here! I'll do anything you want. Please God, let me stay." The thought of my pets wondering where I was, wanting to go outside to use the restroom, needing food and water was overwhelming.

Vickie was my partner of 8 years. We had met when I was new in town and getting over a broken relationship. I disliked Vickie when I first met her. I found her to be too talkative and she had the habit of calling attention to me when I would walk into a room. We eventually developed a friendship that stunningly turned into something more meaningful. She was funny, warm, and had a sense of loyalty and family that I had never experienced before. I thought about someone calling her to let her know I was gone. I thought about the pain it would cause her and I felt a guilty for the position we were in.

I calmly told the paramedic that I felt like closing my eyes and going to sleep but if I did, something bad was going to happen. I asked her if I was going to be okay. She demanded that I keep my eyes open. The tone of her voice changed from being soothing to stern and urgent. I am sure she had heard something like this before because from that moment on she began poking at my leg and yelling for me to stay awake and keep my eyes open.

The paramedic drifted back into the distance and the thoughts in my mind became the only thing I heard again. "God please make me be okay. They need me. I'll help others. I'll do something worthwhile – you name it. I'll be the best person I can be and I'll help people. Please just let me stay. I'll start right away. Please God..." and with that I was jolted back to reality. Everything was loud and bright. Too loud and too bright.

The man that had been demanding my insurance information was now within inches of my face and squeezing my arm. The Paramedic was pushing him off of me and telling him he better sit down. The siren blasted and then stopped. The doors flew open and the freezing cold poured over me. Biting pain washed over my entire body and I let out a gasp. The pain was overwhelming and on a scale of which I have never experienced before – nor since. Agony would have been a welcomed relief.

Tests showed that I had a brain bleed. A concussion was, pardon the pun, a no brainer. My head pounded and the throbbing pain in my body was keeping the same beat. The attending physician neglected to inform me of the risks of such a significant head injury and allowed me to sign on the dotted line and told I could head home. Thankfully the hospital had a cab program that took people home at no cost.

I went to the reception area to wait for the cab. It was here that I ran into the man from the ambulance that was so concerned about my insurance. He was the other driver. I overheard the nurses talking. He had claimed he was injured so he could ride in the ambulance and try to talk to me. He attempted to tell them he was my husband and needed to be in the room with me. Luckily the paramedic was still present and made sure they knew who he was.

When I sat down he instantly came over to me and started demanding to know who my insurance company was. I told him I didn't have anything with me but that a police report was probably done and he could get the information there. He began to shout that he was the victim and he knew his rights. The room began to spin and I felt sick. He told me that he made sure everyone at the accident scene heard his story and I had no chance to play the story any other way. I remember watching him and wondering what possessed someone to be so crazy. My concern at the moment wasn't either vehicle or who was at fault. My concern was getting home and waiting for the pain to stop. Eventually security appeared and escorted him out of the building.

I remained still and waited for the room to stop spinning as people walking by staring at me. The swelling of my head and face was starting to really take on a life of its own. My eye lids felt heavy and I could see my forehead protruding over my eyebrow. I was starting to wonder just how bad I looked when my phone rang.

I answered it but the ringing in my ears made it difficult to hear. I couldn't tell what the other person was saying. Through the pulsing ringing I was able to establish that it was Rick.

Rick was the Director of the agency where I worked. He was a middle age man with big ideas. Rick did wonders for the agency in terms of growth but had a tendency to make emotionally based decisions that crippled the agency as much as his intellectual decisions assisted it. Rick was the kind of guy that would promote those he liked and get rid of those he didn't, regardless of performance. His leadership styled trickled down to the rest of the leadership and it became a mean-girl or high school mentality culture.

Rick heard I was in an accident and wanted to know if I was on my way to work when it happened. I found out later that he and Karen, the District Manager at the time, had been concerned that if I were on my way to work at the time of the accident that the agency could be held liable. He was calling to cover their bases but led me to believe he was calling to check on me yet never once asked if I was alright. He only wanted a clear answer if I was headed to work. When I told him I was taking a friend to the airport he told me "Have a better day" and hung up.

The cab came. Coincidentally, as we approached the very intersection where my accident occurred a few hours before, we were almost struck by a truck that ran the red light. The truck started to slide toward us. I watched out of the passenger window as the truck careened toward me. My heart began to pound and for a moment I felt as though my plea to stay on this earth had been reconsidered. At that very moment the truck hit a patch of dry concrete that threw the vehicle to the side and it came to a halt slamming into the curb next to us. I remember the cab driver laughing and saying "Man that would have sucked for you huh?"

Well, yes it would have.

I went home to my pets. The emptiness of the house seemed even greater and only grew as my body began to stiffen and the swelling reached its peak. I had no one to help take care of me so I called a neighbor that lived behind me and explained that I had been in a car accident and if she didn't see or hear my dogs for a period of time to please check on me. She agreed. I felt better knowing that someone might be aware if I had a problem.

I tried to rest and had a hard time getting comfortable. No matter what position, no matter what side, the pain was unbearable. My body screamed in pain and I couldn't move very well. My head was spinning and my vision dimmed and sharpened with no rhyme or reason. I had feelings of being faint mixed with nausea that I prayed would not result in the need to vomit. The thought of the movements required for that action mixed with the aftermath of pain scared me. I tried to sleep but my dog Meg parked herself next to me and kept digging her nails into my arm. Every time I tried to doze off she woke me up. I was irritated and exhausted. I wanted her to leave me alone but didn't have the strength to do anything about it. I couldn't move my arms away from her and I surely couldn't make her leave the bed.

As the night turned to morning it occurred to me that someone with a head injury needs to have a caretaker to check on them every so often to make sure they are not slipping away. There is no one in the world that can convince me that Meg was not that caretaker for me that night. I believe she saved me because she refused to leave my side and if she did, she stared at me for a long time before she ran to get a drink and then would run back to my side. This annoying dog kept checking on me and likely saved me from slipping away. Meg passed away in January of 2014. I miss her every day.

Though I wasn't healed and shouldn't be driving I went in to work for a few hours over the course of the next week. I suffered from various ailments associated with a major head injury. I suffered from debilitating pain for the better part of a year but continued to work. Missing work was something that wasn't tolerated and despite my condition I knew I had no choice but to be present. I also knew if I said anything to my employer, they would either demote me or terminate me as leave was frowned upon and always faced some sort of consequence. I was required to remain on call 24/7 regardless of any issues and that included medical leave so I did not want to rock that boat.

I eventually recovered with lingering ailments that I suffer with to this day. As I continued to get better, my promise to do anything if I could stay, slowly faded away.

My weight had ballooned to close to 270 pounds. At 5' 5", I was a big girl but never thought to feel bad about my weight and body image until my mid to late thirties when I began working for the agency and was subjected to that high school mean girl mentality.

I had a brief stint with a manager that to date is still the most insecure human being I have ever met. She had an assistant manager that made it a point to talk about my size and lifestyle every chance she had with no consequence. When I told the manager I had my fill of it, I was told that the Assistant was an unhappy person and to take her comments with a grain of salt. I endured the abuse and worked my way to a promotion.

I was promoted to manager of a rough and tumble location. The store was in a rundown part of town known for danger at dusk and the job was very physically demanding. I was given the assignment because Rick said I was the closest thing to a guy he had so he put me there to see if I could make a difference in the failing venture.

Rick always approached me as if I were one of the boys. I'm not sure if he assumed that being gay and a female meant that I wanted to be a boy or if he was just awkward enough to assume that gay females like to be punched on the shoulder and called "sport" every now and then. When he told me that I was the closest thing to a guy he had, I brushed off Rick's comment as ignorance and set sights on turning the location around. The store was full of problem employees who smoked pot in the backroom and smuggled merchandise out of every open door.

Not long after I began leading the store, the problem employees departed and I was eventually fortunate enough to hire a great group of guys that were hard workers and very loyal. They were young men all under the age of 20 and would outwork most of the seasoned adults that came our way. Because of their hard work and dedication the store began to thrive and turn a profit. Something no one at the agency thought was possible.

One afternoon an employee named Joe approached me. Joe was a tall young man hired because Vickie's mother recommended him. He began as an unmotivated 15 year old and turned into one of the best employees I have ever had. "Hey, there's some lady out here going off on everyone. She won't tell me what her problem is. What do you want me to do?" I told him I would go see what was happening.

Little did I know, the antichrist was waiting for me on the other side of the double silver doors.

"Hi, I heard you were upset. What can I do for you?" I said as politely as possible.

"What the fuck do I want with your fat ass? Who the fuck are you? What, you think you can come up to me like you matter and have me think anything of you? Look at your fat ass. I bet you cry yourself to sleep every night over a bucket of ice cream knowing that no one loves you. You're a pathetic loser you fat ass bitch." She spit beads of venom as she spoke. I took a step back.

"I'm sorry, I should have introduced myself. My name is Laura and I am the Store Manager. I was told you were upset and came out to see what had happened and how I could fix the issue." I said again as politely as possible.

"YOUR fat ass wants to help ME? BITCH GET THE FUCK AWAY FROM ME! You are so fat I swear to GOD I can smell you from here. Why don't you go kill yourself and do the world a fucking favor? We don't need another FAT ASS in this world. ESPECIALLY some Rosie O'Donnell fat piece of shit thinking she is running something like you have a brain in your fucking head. Get the FUCK away from me while I do my thing!" she continued to spit while she talked but I remained a safe shower free distance from her. I contemplated having her leave but knew if I told my leadership that I had a customer leave the location, I would be reprimanded. I opted to walk away as my presence was clearly making matters worse.

"That's right fat Rosie bitch, waddle your fat ass away!"

I was steaming and felt trapped. I couldn't ask her to leave and I didn't want her at my location. It was a no win situation. I left the floor and went to the production area. I called the front and told Joe to let me know if there were any other problems.

Within a few minutes I was paged to the front of the store. As I came up the isle I heard the same woman spewing racial insults at people of her own race as well as the race of those around her.

As I approached she began hurling insults at me again. "Oh here comes the fat faggot! What are you going to do you fat Rosie bitch? Didn't I tell you to go kill yourself in a ditch and put yourself out of everyone else's misery? Fuck sake you fat ass, put down the donuts and start saying NO to lard, you fat fuck!"

Joe approached me looking sad. "I'm sorry Laura. I didn't want to call you up here because of the things she is saying to you but I can't get her to check out and I can't get her to leave the store. She just wants to yell at everyone."

"That's right you big taco bean, run to the fat ass. You two deserve each other!"

Now I was mad.

"You little river runners slither into our country and take over and think I owe you something well fuck you!"

"Joe, take the other employees into the back. You don't need to put up with her. I'll take care of it from here." I said quietly. I was boiling but determined to be professional.

"You sure Laura? She's a huge bitch" Joe said, looking back.

"Yep, I'm sure. None of you deserve to put up with her. Go in the back and I'll take care of it."

As Joe walked away my anger exploded when she called him another name. It is one thing to attack me but to attack these young men who have done nothing to her, that was the final straw. I knew my decision would be met with some sort of negative response from the leadership at my agency and frankly, I didn't care.

I turned around to this woman who was still spewing her hatred in every direction possible and for a moment, I thought about grabbing her and forcefully leading her out of the store but that is assault. I wouldn't be drawn to her level.

"Ma'am, I'm not sure what your issue is but at this point, you can leave the store on your own or I can call the police who will escort you out. Either way, you will not stay here any longer."

"What the fuck are YOU going to do about it tubs? You gonna chase me? Ohhhhh....IIIIIII get it. You want to fuck me! Yeah, you wish you lesbian faggot bitch. I would slit my wrists before I'd lower myself to something like you. You eat McDonalds every day don't you bitch? Well you can keep steppin and get someone who isn't a lowly Mexican, African, fat ass Queer or Lilly White KKK Mother Fucker out here to wait on me because I aint doin' SHIT with any of you fuckers and I AINT leavin'!"

"I'm sorry, you are now no longer welcome at this or any other location. We do not need nor want people that speak or think like you in our stores so at this time you need to leave this store - now."

"Oh! People like me huh? I get it you racist bitch! Yeah, you don't LIKE me because of what I look like! You're a stupid fat queer cunt bitch and you'll have to pick me up and MAKE me leave and IF you EVEN think about touching me – I am going to kick your fat ass up and down these isles so when you're ready to go – LETS GO!"

"I will give you until the count of five to remove yourself from the store before I call the police and have you removed."

"Fuck you!"

"1"

"Eat ass bitch!"

"2"

"Lick it queer bitch!"

"3"

"Eeeewwww I'm SO scared of you. Fat faggot bitch!"

I pick up the phone and start to dial.

"4"

She begins walking toward the door as the other customers circled around her. A screaming match broke out between her and two or three of the other regular customers. They screamed at her to leave and she screamed various racially explicit insults at them.

I continue to dial 9-1-1 because my desire to have her leave the store was now overshadowed by my concern that she was circled by a group of people and may actually be injured because of her big mouth.

"9-1-1 do you need police or medical?"

"Police right away"

"What is happening?"

"I have customer who is starting fights with people and is currently circled by them. She could be hurt. We need an officer here right away."

The dispatcher asked me for a description and various other information. They told me to watch for the officers and remain at a safe distance from the situation.

The crazy woman walked back toward me and demanded to make her purchase. I refused and told her calmly "I explained this to you. You have passed the point of being able to purchase in this or any of our other locations. You need to leave the store immediately. Police have been dispatched and you need to leave."

"So they cops are comin'. I don't give a shit. You are still fat, stupid and a queer. Nothing is going to change that!"

She began walking toward the door still hurling insults at me and the customers trying to get her to stop talking. I walked with her toward the door. Not because I wanted the "power" of having her leave but because I was afraid one of the customers may hit her as she walked away. I walked her to the door to protect her yet she continued to hurl insults my way.

As she stepped outside she told me "You just want to walk me out so you can look at my fine tight ass. That's right you queer bitch, look all you want honey because there aint nothing in these pants that want any part of some fat piece of shit like YOU so – watch me walk away honey because my ass is the finest thing a faggot like you will EVER see!"

I felt a great sense of relief as she departed. The mob of customers congregated at the front of the store began to disperse and as they did, several came up to me and apologized for the things she said to me. As I made my way through the crowd and walked toward my office I began to crack.

Rage over the way she talked to my staff and the customers consumed me. I was ashamed that I allowed her to remain in the store as long as I did because I feared being reprimanded by the executives of my agency. I should have thrown those concerns out and done what was right for my employees and customers. I should have worried about the consequences later.

I entered my office and began to type out the incident report that I knew my company would want. There was a knock at the door. The police were there and wanted a statement and description. As I spoke to them I noticed that one of them had a great resemblance to my father and I melted. Tears started rolling down my cheek as I relayed the things that had happened and the things that were said. Had this officer not reminded me so much of my father, who was also a cop, I would have probably been fine. His presence reminded me of times as a child that I would call my father to sort out the various traumas of my childhood. It was the safety, understanding and strength that only a dad can provide.

The officer came around the desk and put his hand on my shoulder. "You didn't deserve any of that and I can tell you that in my line of work, I hear all kinds of things tossed my way. I don't like it but eventually you have to have pity on the people that need to stoop to those levels. This wasn't about you at all. She probably came in here looking for a fight and if it was not here, it would have been the business next door or up the street. I am going to find her and make sure she knows she can't step foot in this building again. My advice, for what it's worth, take a few minutes. Get the emotion out and then pull yourself together and be there for your employees. You all had a rough time today and they'll need you to be strong so give yourself some time to feel it and then brush it off and help them do the same. This is just one crazy acting like a fool. Nothing more."

With that, he and the other officer set off to ban what would become known as "The Mouth of the South".

As they shut the door behind them I knew I needed to call my direct supervisor. As I relayed the incident to my boss Kevin, emotion began to well and my voice started to crack. Kevin was a laid back kind of guy. Kevin was in his thirties and had been a cop once. He was pretty unflappable and I appreciated his style. He was a hands off supervisor who allowed me to make the decisions that needed to be made while supporting me all the way but in this moment, he knew something was very wrong. I couldn't finish the story, I had to hang up and as I did so, the emotion exploded.

I sobbed in rage, disappointment, embarrassment and despair. I felt that if I were not as fat as I was, this person would not have had the ammunition to continue her rant. I was angry with my executives because I should have been afforded the latitude to expel someone from my location who behaved in a racist and demeaning way without fear of consequence. Mostly I felt responsible for this terrible human being attacking my staff and customers. Guilt consumed me. It took me the better part of an hour to pull myself together. Instead of calling Kevin back, I sent him an email to explain the situation because each time I began to pick up the phone, my emotions began pouring forward.

Once I pulled myself together I went to the production area and called the staff back. I apologized to them for the customers' ignorance and reminded each of them how fantastic they were. I explained to these young men that sometimes people, no matter how young or old, behave poorly and blame others. I addressed the woman's racial rants and told my staff that they never have to put up with someone speaking to them the way this woman spoke and if they ever encountered someone doing such, they were to walk away immediately and get me. "There isn't enough money on this planet for you to have to endure someone talking to you that way. You do not get paid to be abused."

Their response?

These young men of various ethnic background, many of which were still in high school or taking GED classes, these young men who were not even 19 or 20 years old said to me "We don't care what she said to us Laura. We are sorry she said those things to you and just so you know, YOU don't make enough for someone to talk to you that way. We think you should have kicked her ass." I was stunned. These guys were even more amazing than I thought.

"I'm sorry I came and got you Laura. I should have just handled it on my own because if I didn't tell you about it, you wouldn't have gone out there and she wouldn't have said those things to you." Joe's voice waivered as he spoke and he stared at the floor.

My heart melted. These young men knew more about humanity than many of the adults I knew then or know now. I made sure Joe knew nothing was his fault and worked hard to raise the spirits of the store. I couldn't outwardly dwell on it because these guys would follow my lead and as much as I hated that woman for the things she said to them, I wasn't about to allow her the power to control our environment after her departure.

I toiled about the incident for days. I had flashbacks of her insults toward my employees and me. As my boss sat across from me uncomfortably conveying the executive's predictable dissatisfaction that I allowed this unruly person to remain in the store – he acknowledged that had I removed her, the same discussion would have been happening for that. I was in a no win situation and we both knew it.

"No matter what I do, they seem to find fault. If I weave I should jump. If I jump I should weave."

"You're absolutely right." Kevin said. "You just have to do the best you can and I'll keep running interference every chance I get."

I fell into a deep depression for quite some time. I wanted to look for another job but felt that I was unemployable. My leadership made sure I knew I was replaceable. They worked hard to ensure I felt the sting of exclusion and bewilderment of contempt.

My co-workers would only call me on a landline. They didn't want my number to appear on their cell phone bills and would joke about me being on an island by myself. They would marvel at my treatment but also made sure to keep a safe distance during manager meetings for fear of retaliation.

My self-esteem was at an all-time low. One night Vickie was watching a television show. There was a car chase. As the tires on the television squealed and the suspects' car flipped over ending in a predictable crash, the room spun. I flashed back to my accident. I was IN the accident. My memory flashed through the scenes I could remember of the accident and came to a halt on the memory of me being in the back of the ambulance begging God to let me stay on this earth. When the realization hit me that I made a promise and had done nothing to honor it, the flashback disappeared and I was left swaying in my living room upset and full of guilt and disappointment in myself.

I made a promise and forgot about it? What was wrong with me? I was given the ability to take care of my pets just like I asked for and then I failed to even attempt to fulfill my promise. I was ashamed and determined to do what I said I would do.

I made the decision to lose weight to enhance my self-esteem. The woman that said all of those horrible things continued to haunt me and I used her as well as the horrible people I worked for as motivation to stick to the plan. I had no idea where to start but was going to figure something out.

I decided to call the local YMCA to see if they had personal trainers. I had exhausted all other avenues and because of my size, no trainer would take me for fear I was going to drop dead. I was put in touch with a woman named Jessica who ran the fitness programs. I explained the situation to her and she suggested I join boot camp. I was fearful I couldn't do it but she assured me I would be fine. I signed up for camp that day and began to prepare for the following Monday's start date.

I went home that night and announced to my family that I would be taking the classes, eating right and losing weight. Vickie had her doubts but encouraged me to do it.

The next night I came home to not 1 but 3 freshly baked goods from my list of favorites. I refused to eat any of them and after a lengthy argument with Vickie – I embarked upon a journey that would unknowingly lead me to my promise.

The first day of boot camp was testing. I completed it and thought "I've got this!" I had always known that I was overweight but also had a long history as a child and young adult of being very fit and active. I called myself "Fat but fit".

The second day of boot camp the group ran downtown. As I lagged behind I felt like I was wearing a lead suit. I couldn't keep up and the group disappeared. I had to stop and walk and as I did, reality came crashing down around me.

My failure to keep up unleashed a flurry demeaning internal dialogue. "I'm not fit at all. I am just fat. I am EXACTLY what that evil woman said I was. I AM a fat ass. I can't keep up and I should be able to. I am nothing but a fat ass!" I was disgusted and felt utter and completely defeated.

I struggled to catch my breath while my body fought every step. Just as I was preparing to turn around and leave, Jessica appeared. She was the boot camp instructor and had come back to check on me.

As we walked she asked me how I was. My voice cracked. I was upset. I told her that I always thought I was fit but realized at that moment I was very heavy and very out of shape and didn't think I could do the class.

Jessica listened and walked next to me. She asked if she could tell me her story. I agreed. I knew I wasn't going to be back but didn't want to be rude and embarrass myself by walking away.

"I was overweight and decided to change my life. I became a personal trainer in my quest for knowledge about my own body and my own program. I learned what needed to be done and I worked at it. It wasn't easy but if I can do it, so can you."

I told her I appreciated her talking with me. She said she had to get back to the front of the group and asked if I was okay. I told her I was and as she began to run away, she turned, jogging backwards and said "You know Laura, not all trainers start out thin." And with that, she ran to the top of the hill and disappeared.

Jessica's statement has been a driving force in my life from the moment she spoke them.

That night I had a Tim McGraw and Faith Hill concert to attend and missed the normal 6:00 A.M. class the next day. The next afternoon I received an email from the Director of the YMCA. Her name was Judy and she was reaching out to me to find out if I was coming back to class. She expressed concern that I hadn't returned and wanted me to promise to meet her the next morning for class.

We exchanged a few emails. I explained my absence and promised to attend class the next day. From that moment on Jessica and Judy became my personal cheerleaders.

I finished boot camp and didn't lose a bunch of weight but did become considerably more fit. Through the four week session I pushed myself to run a little bit further and try a little bit harder each day. I also started working out on the days between the program. I eventually moved from the back of the pack to the front. The first time I finished a run as the first one back I spent a few minutes enjoying my victory. I looked up and saw Jessica smiling at me. "It feels kind of good to pass everyone, doesn't it? You've come so far. Aren't you glad you didn't quit?" I was embarrassed for a split second. I never wanted to take pride in placing someone else in a lesser than position than I was but for sporting purposes, I had to admit that I felt pretty good about it. There were a few women in the class that expressed irritation that those of us that couldn't keep up were holding the class back. Now they were the ones I passed by as they struggled. I felt a sense of accomplishment. Anyone who has been significantly overweight and improved their fitness levels understands what that moment meant. It was not about those women rather the "I can't" they represent. I was able to overcome "I can't" and excel. I allowed myself to bask in pride for a while. I earned it.

Eventually Jessica left the YMCA and I continued on my path. There were very few very overweight people at the gym and I made the commitment to go no matter what. Eventually a personal training test was offered by an accredited agency and coincidentally, it was being held at the YMCA I frequented so I enrolled. I was struggling with my weight loss program because I lacked the knowledge to do anything other than run on a treadmill and lift some weights. Nutrition, hydration, sleep and overall fitness were nothing I had been exposed to so I enrolled to enhance my own efforts. Again, not knowing that doing so would be another step in fulfilling my promise.

I passed the test and was awarded a Personal Trainer certification. I mounted it and hung it I my living room with pride. The new coordinator for the YMCA that took Jessica's place gave me a call. Angela had been told to contact me because Judy felt I had something to offer the YMCA. As someone that was well over 220 pounds, I could be a role model and the fact that I was a certified trainer and active in meeting my goals was intriguing to Judy.

Angela was a young and very sweet person who wanted good things for everyone. She was extremely knowledgeable and worked hard to present programs that would appeal to the masses. She allowed me to work for the YMCA and was instrumental in my development there.

I eventually started running the very boot camp that I had started at. I also started seeing clients on an individual basis and enjoyed the challenge of finding activities that matched the abilities of my clients. Many of my first clients are still with me today and while some have moved to other states and gone on to great things, I value each and every one of them. My clientele list has grown over the years and while some have been taken from this earth entirely too early while others have moved on to other programs, each and every person helped form the trainer I am today.

Angela nominated me for and I won a prestigious award through the YMCA. I was flown to the YMCA National Convention in Salt Lake City Utah and was recognized for my unique programs and commitment to community change.

Soledad O'Brien was the keynote speaker and very complementary toward me when we met after the event. She and Vickie hit it off and traded shopping secrets regarding shoes and current styles. We had the chance to take a photo with her and I shied away but with Soledad's encouragement telling me "Get in here! I want to have MY picture taken with YOU! You are amazing!" I relented. She was very genuine and warm and I enjoyed meeting her.

The event as a whole was very overwhelming and contrary to everything about my personality. I am pretty low key and like to do well but prefer to be low key with occasional brief appearances on radar. I don't want to fly completely under the radar but do prefer it the majority of the time. The weekend presented itself very differently. I was asked to sign napkins and stopped throughout my visit to talk about my weight loss, me and my outlook on fitness. I was invited to various cities across the country to come and speak at facilities or groups. I remember turning to Vickie several times for a reality check. "Is this real? I don't get it. It's just me."

And before I could finish my sentence we would be approached by another person wanting introduce themselves. It was a memory I'll carry throughout my life because there are not many times in a normal everyday life that people want your autograph unless you are signing a credit card receipt at the store. I am still honored and value that time in my life.

As I have matured as a trainer my philosophies have changed. When I began training I pushed the envelope. I engaged in the hardcore off the charts training programs. I invented workouts that were designed to push the human body to the limits while improving cardiorespiratory function seemingly by the minute. I engaged in each and every one of my workouts. If I could do it – so could my clients. If I couldn't – I kept at it until I could and then I implemented the exercise in a program.

My approach now is aimed at long-term compliance and success. Anyone can engage in extreme fitness for a short period of time but the body is not designed to be under a constant state of physical stress any more than it is designed to be under a constant state of psychological stress. Eventually each system will begin to implode. That is when injuries and ailments begin to appear and that is not what I wanted for my clients.

We need to physically push ourselves to the brink on occasion to show our minds and bodies that anything is possible but it is the daily steps that create and maintain our progress.

In the following pages you will find fitness programs, meal plans and recipes. Like trying on a pair of shoes, not one size fits all and any responsible trainer would make sure a client was aware of that fact from the start. When I am training a client, I am with them for 1 to 4 hours a week. It is the other 20 or 23 hours in the week that make or break a plan.

I am constantly asked how one can succeed. How one can finally meet the goals they set as a resolution. My response will always be the same. Consistency. You have to want it bad enough to follow your plan no matter what. If you are just starting out or returning from time off from fitness you have to take baby steps. Your body demands it and if anyone tells you otherwise, find another source for information. Our bodies need time to adjust to a different activity level. Without proper conditioning we fall victim to injury, ailments or worse. Give your body time to learn what you want from it and it will support you throughout your journey.

As you read through the information and create the fitness and meal plans that work for you, always be mindful of your ultimate goal. Is it fitness as a whole? Is it cardio improvement or weight loss? Whatever the goal, keep it on the "front page" of your life. The more you think about it the more successful you will be.

Let's get started!

2 THE BEGINNING

The first thing one needs to do is establish with your physician if working out and changing nutrition is a good idea. NEVER start a fitness program without consulting a medical provider. This needs to be done first.

Assuming the instructions above were followed - let's get started!

From this point forward I will lead you through the steps to better nutrition and better fitness. It is up to you to execute the plan and stick to it. Remember – if you want it bad enough – you'll do it!

It's time to test your fitness level! Dress in appropriate workout attire. You should have shoes that fit properly and are laced to provide maximum support and comfortable. If you prefer shorts, this is the time to pick out your favorite pair and match them with your favorite workout shirt. These are the clothes I want you to write down and remember because this is what you were wearing when you embarked on the program that will help you achieve your goals!

You need to have water available for your workout and be prepared to sweat! If you are under the misconception that you need to avoid drinking while you workout – change that philosophy now. Your body needs the water to stay healthy.

3 FITNESS TESTING

The first thing I want you to do is establish your resting heart rate. Your resting heart rate is exactly how it sounds. It is a count of how many times your heart beats while at rest. Your heart rate fluctuates throughout the day so the goal here is to establish a baseline number for where your heart rate sits when you are not active.

Here is how to do it:

o Get a good night's sleep for 5 days in a row
o Each morning upon waking and BEFORE you get out of bed – measure your heart rate.
o Watch the clock
o Start on an easy to remember number
o Place your index finger on your wrist and locate your heart beat. (This method is preferred over placing your finger on the artery in your neck)
o Start your count on your preferred number. Each beat is one and independent of the clock. Do not count the seconds of the clock. Only count the beats of your heart.
o Do this for one full minute
o Write down the day and the number
o Repeat for 5 days

At the end of 5 days add all of the days together and divide by 5. This is your average resting heart rate.

EXAMPLE:

Jenny is determining her resting heart rate. She keeps a pen and paper by the bed with the days of the week written down ahead of time. (Jenny does this because when she wakes up she is groggy and doesn't want to rely on her sleepy memory to determine what day it is!)

At the end of the week Jenny reviews her record.

Monday – 55   Thursday – 56
Tuesday – 48   Friday - 58
Wednesday – 61

Jenny adds all of the numbers together and writes 278 down. (Hint: I recommend that you double check your math just to be sure you are accurate.)

Jenny divides 278 by 5 and gets 55.6. For all purposes I round up so I would say Jenny has a resting heart rate of 56 beats per minute. Not bad Jenny! Congratulations!

According to the National Institute of Health, the average resting heart rate for children 10 years and older, and adults (including seniors) is 60 - 100 beats per minute. Well-trained athletes is 40 - 60 beats per minute.

My resting heart rate has been as low as 42 during peak training and as high as 56 during my time off from training. If your resting heart rate is higher than the established norm, my suggestion would be that you talk to your physician. Everyone has different "norms" and if they are okay with it – carry on!

Resting heart rate – DONE. On to the fun stuff!

First things first – warm up!

Here are some options. Feel free to adjust them for mobility or restrictions as needed. The goal is to warm up the muscles and organs so your body knows it is time to workout and cooperates!

Warm Up Options for 10 minutes

1. Briskly walking on the treadmill and a slight incline if tolerated
2. Lay down on the floor face down and get back up
3. Jump rope at a slow steady pace
4. Walk the stairs
5. Jump squats
6. Push-ups followed by jumping jacks
7. Jumping jacks at a slow to medium pace

Take 2 minutes to rest and have a sip of water. Are you ready? Let's go!

Fitness Testing

Get a pen and paper. Write the date and time down. Write down what you are wearing and it would be a good idea to write your starting weight, measurements for your biceps, chest, waist, hips and thighs. These are, of course, your starting numbers and something you will value as you progress. Write down each testing activity and how you chose to complete it (modified or standard).

Tools you will need for all tests:

o   Your pen and paper
o   Ruler
o   Duct tape
o   Metronome (If you don't have one there are tons of free apps out there. Set it to 96 beats per minute)
o   A STURDY 12 inch step, bench or box. It should be able to hold your weight
o   A stop watch or timer that can measure a full minute that can be easily read
o   Someone to help you run the stop watch, count and urge you on - if you so choose
o   A chair

The Push Up Test

This test is to measure your strength and endurance.

Tools:
o   Pen and paper
o   Stop Watch
o   Friend to run the watch and count if you wish

Here is how to do it:

o   The timer starts when your push-ups start. If you are alone, keep the timer close.
o   Your goal is to lower your chest at least three inches from the floor. If this is too low, do the absolute best you can. Remember – this is the starting point!
o   For one full minute – do as many push-ups as you can, as fast as you can!

(Hint: Watch your form. Your butt should be lower than your shoulders when you start. As you lower to a push up, your shoulders should drop to the same level as your hips. At no time should you look like you are bobbing for apples! Elbows bend, shoulders and chest lower, hips go too!)

At the end of the minute, write your number down and then enjoy the rest that should not be any longer than 3 minutes.

Compare yourself against American College of Sports Medicine's standards while you regain your strength.

MEN:

	20-29	30-39	40-49	50-59	60+
Excellent	> 54	> 44	> 39	> 34	> 29
Good	45-54	35-44	30-39	25-34	20-29
Average	35-44	24-34	20-29	15-24	10-19
Poor	20-34	15-24	12-19	8-14	5-9
Very Poor	< 20	< 15	< 12	< 8	< 5

WOMEN:

	20-29	30-39	40-49	50-59	60+
Excellent	>48	>39	>34	>29	>19
Good	34-48	25-39	20-34	15-29	5-19
Average	17-33	12-24	8-19	6-14	3-4
Poor	6-16	4-11	3-7	2-5	1-2
Very Poor	< 6	< 4	< 3	< 2	< 1

Remember – if your level is not where you think or want it to be – YOU can change that. It is why you bought this book!

On to the next test!

The Crunch Test

This test is to measure your abdominal strength and endurance

Tools:

- o   Pen and Paper
- o   Stop Watch
- o   Friend to run the watch and count
- o   Ruler
- o   Duct Tape

Here is how to do it:

- o   The timer starts when your crunches start. If you are alone, keep the timer close.
- o   Your goal is to do as many crunches in one minute as you can.

There are specific guidelines I want you to follow for these crunches.
Lie on your back with your hips and shoulders aligned. Bend your knees and keep your feet flat on the floor. Your heels should be about 18 inches away from your butt while your palms are lying flat on the floor with your hands open and palms flat and next to your hips.

Place the ruler next to your fingertips. Take note of where your fingertips rest while in this position and then mark 6 inches further as your goal spot. When I complete this testing for my clients, I place a piece of duct tape on the floor to mark the spot I want them to hit during each crunch. You will only count the crunches that meet that mark. If you fall short, it does not count.

For general testing you do not have to measure your reach but it is advisable if you want measurable results with no room for doubt.

(Hint: Watch your form! Your hands stay on the floor sliding toward the goal line during each crunch. This is a must! Engage your abs and lift your shoulders off the floor. Your head should stay aligned with your shoulders. Bobbing your head forward and backward is stressful on neck muscles. If your shoulders rise, your head should rise with them. If your shoulders lower, your head should lower with them.)

Do as many proper crunches as you can in one minute. While you take a short (no longer than 3 minutes) rest – compare yourself against American College of Sports Medicine's standards.

MEN:

Rating	< 35 years	35-44 years	> 45 years
Excellent	60	50	40
Good	45	40	25
Marginal	30	25	15
Needs Work	15	10	5

WOMEN:

Rating	< 35 years	35-44 years	> 45 years
Excellent	50	40	30
Good	40	25	15
Marginal	25	15	10
Needs Work	10	6	4

This is your starting number. We will check this again in a month. You will make sure you see improvement in those numbers!

NEXT!

3 Minute Step Test

This test measures your cardiovascular fitness level.

Tools:

- o   Pen and paper
- o   Stop watch
- o   Metronome
- o   12" step
- o   Chair to rest in after test
- o   Friend to help keep track of time and take your pulse if you wish

Here is how to do it:

- o   Set the metronome or metronome app to 96 beats per minute
- o   Face the step (needs to be able to hold your weight and as absolute close to 12" high as possible. This is a MUST!)
- o   Start the metronome
- o   The stop watch starts when your stepping starts
- o   For each click of the metronome, you should be taking one step.
- o   Do this for 3 full minutes
- o   After the 3 minutes, immediately sit down and take your pulse for one full minute. Record this number.

Here is an example:

Roberta is doing the 3 minute step test while Carmen times her and then will take her blood pressure after the test is complete.

Roberta starts the metronome and starts to step. Click, Click, Click, Click. Roberta repeats to herself. Up, Up, Down, Down. Up, Up, Down, Down. She does this as she steps up with her left foot and then steps up with her right foot. She steps down with her left foot and steps down with her right foot. Up, Up, Down, Down.

Carmen tells Roberta when she has 10 seconds left on the timer. "Stop and Sit" Carmen commands. Roberta complies and holds out her arm. Carmen takes Roberta's pulse and writes the number down on Roberta's record.

(Hint: Take a practice run and briefly get the tempo and stepping down. Many people try to do the entire sequence with each and every click and that is not correct. Each click represents a step. One step.)

Time to take a short 3 minute rest and compare yourself against the YMCA standards.

Men:

	18-25	26-35	36-45	46-55	56-65	65+
Excellent	50-76	51-76	49-76	56-82	60-77	59-81
Good	79-84	79-85	80-88	87-93	86-94	87-92
Above Average	88-93	88-94	92-88	95-101	97-100	94-102
Average	95-100	96-102	100-105	103-111	103-109	104-110
Below Average	102-107	104-110	108-113	113-119	111-117	114-118
Poor	111-119	114-121	116-124	121-126	119-128	121-126
Very Poor	124-157	126-161	130-163	131-159	131-154	130-151

Women:

	18-25	26-35	36-45	46-55	56-65	65+
Excellent	52-81	58-80	51-84	63-91	60-92	70-92
Good	85-93	85-92	89-96	95-101	97-103	96-101
Above Average	96-102	95-101	100-104	104-110	106-111	104-111
Average	104-110	104-110	107-112	113-118	113-118	116-121
Below Average	113-120	113-119	115-120	120-124	119-127	123-126
Poor	122-131	122-129	124-132	126-132	129-135	128-133
Very Poor	135-169	134-171	137-169	137-171	141-174	135-155

Write down your results and prepare to see these numbers change!

If the step test is not something you can do then you will default to the next test. Feel free to complete this test in conjunction with the others if you are able. Give yourself about 3 minutes to recover and then get started!

1 Mile Walking Test

This test measures your cardiovascular fitness level.

Tools:

- o Stop Watch
- o One measured exact flat mile
    - o School track (if it is quarter mile track then 4 laps are a mile)
    - o Neighborhood route (measured in car)
    - o Treadmill

The watch starts when your mile starts. Get through your mile as fast as you can. Write the number down and congratulate yourself. Your testing is complete!

Fitness Testing – DONE! On to the plan!

4 THE PLAN

Creating a plan to follow is the most difficult part of a program. You want to add in activity that you can do, that is beneficial and that yields the results you are looking for.

You are fee to mix and match the following exercises to create your own plan.

Tools:

o   Pen and paper if you wish to create your own plan

Exercises

These exercises are to be done Monday – Wednesday – Friday Weeks 1, 3 and 5

WARM UP – 10 minutes – see the list from Fitness Testing

Plank Twist – 3 sets of 12-15
To add difficulty – do 3 sets of 20
   o   Get into a push up position
   o   Keep your hands aligned with your shoulders
   o   Legs need to be straight. No knee bend
   o   Feet together
   o   You should be on the balls of our feet
   o   Rotate your torso to one side so your hips are facing the wall
   o   Keep your hands on the floor
   o   Bring your bottom knee in toward the opposite armpit.
   o   Get back into the starting position
   o   Repeat the process with the opposite knee

Skaters – 3 sets of 30 seconds to 1 minute as tolerated. Perform at an 8 out of 10 difficulty.
To make it more difficult – add a hop and/or toe touch your hand to the opposite foot.

- o Start with your feet together
- o Think ice or roller skating here.
- o Step to the left with your left foot
- o Kick your right foot behind
- o Step to the right with your right foot
- o Kick your left foot behind

Dumbbell Bicep Curl – 3 sets of 12-15
To make this exercise effective choose a dumbbell that is an 8 out of 10 difficulty. You want a weight that challenges you but does not compromise form.

- o Stand upright. Feet are shoulder width apart with your knees slightly bent.
- o Place a dumbbell in each hand, palms facing the ceiling with elbows locked against your side.
- o Curl arms toward your face. Stop ¾ of the way up.
- o Pause for a second squeezing your bicep.
- o Slowly lower your arms to the starting position but not all the way down. You want to keep tension on the muscle.

Mountain Climbers – 3 sets of 30 seconds to 1 minute. Push yourself to do the minute!
To make this more difficult extend your time by one minute

- o Start in a push up position with your feet about hip width apart. Keep your butt lower than your shoulders.
- o Bring your knee forward toward the same side elbow
- o Return that foot back to the starting point
- o Bring your opposite knee toward the same side elbow
- o Return that foot back to the starting point
- o Repeat

Windshield Wipers – 3 sets of 12 – 15

- o Lie face up on your back
- o Raise your legs directly above your hips and keep your knees straight
- o Place your arms straight out like you are forming the letter T
- o Place your palms on the ground
- o Slower lower your legs evenly toward your right side. Get as close to the floor without touching it as you can. Be mindful of any pains. If you feel pain – stop!
- o Slowly raise your legs back to the starting position
- o Slowly lower your legs evenly toward your left side. Get as close to the floor without touching it as you can. Stop if you feel pain!

Dumbbell Tricep Extensions – 3 sets of 15

- o Sit or stand with a dumbbell in each hand.
- o Feet shoulder width apart
- o Raise arms to place dumbbells directly over your head
- o Bend your arms slowly moving the weight behind your head being careful not to hit your head
- o Lower the dumbbells until you feel a comfortable stretch on the back of your arms
- o Raise the weights slowly back to the starting position
- o Repeat

V Flys – 3 sets of 15

- o Stand up straight
- o Feet shoulder width apart
- o Arms at your side
- o Palms facing the ceiling
- o Raise your arms from your side to the front even with your chin
- o Raise and lower your arms slowly

Squatting Skater – 3 sets of 12 – 15

o Balance on a leg. Bend forward at the waist extending your arms in front of you and shoulder height
o Extend your opposite foot behind you and point your toe toward the ground locking your knee
o Slowly bend your foundation leg (the leg your standing on) slowly dropping down as low as you can go being mindful not to allow your foundation knee to lean past your foundation toe.
o Hold for a count of 1 second (increase the hold to make this exercise more difficult)
o Slowly raise back to the starting position.
o Complete all reps on the same side before moving to the opposite leg

Overhead one leg chair pose – 3 sets of 12 – 15

o Stand with your feet just slightly apart
o Straighten your arms overhead, lock your elbows and extend your hands as if reaching out to someone
o Bring your shoulders down to their natural position
o Bend at the waist as if you are going to sit in a chair
o Lean on one leg and extend the other slightly in front of you
o Hold for the count of 3 (extend your count to make this more difficult)
o Straighten your stance
o Repeat

**These exercises are to be done Thursday and Saturday
Weeks 1, 3 and 5**

WARM UP – 10 minutes – see the list from Fitness Testing

Jumping Jacks – 3 sets of 1 minute, rest 30 seconds and then 2 sets of 2 minutes

- o Jumping jacks as fast as possible with form in mind
- o Raise arms all the way to the top of your head
- o Lower arms to your side
- o Your job is to do as many jumping jacks as you can
- o To make this exercise more difficult, extend the time, leap higher and faster

Burpy – 3 sets of 1 minute, rest 30 seconds and then 2 sets of 2 minutes

- o Stand up straight with feet hip width apart
- o Lower to the ground into a squat
- o Place your hands palms down on the floor
- o Kick your feet back so that you are in a push up position
- o Jump your feet forward bending at the knee so you are back into a squat position
- o Leap from this position into a jump
- o Repeat
- o To make this exercise more difficult, increase your time and each time you jump attempt to beat the height of the last time

Squat Jack – 3 sets of 1 minute
This is much like a jumping jack but you will be in a squat instead

- o Take a squat position
- o Complete jumping jacks remaining in the squat position
- o Do not come out of the squat position
- o Repeat
- o To make this exercise more difficult – increase your time and speed being mindful of your form

Standing Mountain Climber – 3 sets of 1 minute
This is like climbing a ladder

- o Place a dumbbell in each hand
- o Palms should be facing your body
- o Raise one hand toward the ceiling
- o Raise the opposite leg toward the ceiling at the same time
- o Do not lower your hand any lower than your shoulder
- o Raise your knee as high as your hips
- o Switch position and repeat
- o Continue "climbing" the ladder
- o Push the dumbbells to the ceiling with power
- o To make this difficult more difficult use heavier weights that allow you to keep good form, extend the time and increase the number of sets

**These exercises are to be done Monday – Wednesday – Friday
Weeks 2, 4 and 6**

WARM UP – 10 minutes – see the list from Fitness Testing

Crunching Twist – 3 sets of 20

- o Get into a crunch position
- o Place a hand behind your head
- o Place opposite hand on your stomach
- o Do not pull on your neck when you crunch
- o Crunch up and twist your torso to the opposite knee of the arm behind your head
- o Lower back to the floor
- o Repeat

Extended Plant – 3 sets of 1 minute

- o Get into a plank position
- o Walk your hands forward as far out as you can without compromising your form.
- o Keep your back straight and your abs tight
- o To make this exercise more difficult – extend your time and/or move your hands closer together

Tricep Dip – 3 sets of 12-15

- o Stand with your back to a chair or bench that will not slide and will hold your weight
- o Place your hands on the chair or bench and extend your legs in front of you. Bend your knees for easier (ONLY if needed) or extend and lock your knees for more difficulty
- o Keeping your elbows stuck to your sides
- o Bend your arms to slowly dip your body
- o Do not fall to the ground
- o Dip until your arms are even with the ground
- o If you feel pain, stop

Scorpion Push Up – 3 sets of 12-15

- o Get into a push up position
- o Lower into a push up and bring a leg across the back of your body as if you are trying to touch your heel to the opposite butt cheek
- o Return your leg to the starting position
- o Raise back to a push up
- o Repeat with opposite leg
- o To make this exercise more difficult – extend the sets to 5 and pause as you move your leg to the back. Hold for a count of 5.

Frog Legs – 3 sets of 15

- o Lie face down on a sturdy bench with your torso laying fully supported on the bench
- o Hug the bench tight to give your body stability
- o Bend your knees as if kneeling
- o Extend your legs straight out behind you with your feet touching
- o Repeat in a slow and controlled motion
- o To make this exercise more difficult increase the sets to 5 and place a hold time of 3-5 seconds after extending your legs

Deadlift – 3 sets of 12-15

- o Stand with feet slightly apart with your knees slightly bent
- o Place a dumbbell in each hand with your palms facing behind you
- o Bend at the waist keeping your back flat
- o Pull your shoulders back
- o Suck your belly button in toward your spine
- o Tip your hips back slightly
- o Slowly bend forward at your waist
- o Lower the dumbbells until your torso is just about level with the floor
- o Slowly raise your torso back to the starting position
- o Keep the dumbbells close to your legs/shins as you raise and lower

Alternating or Traveling Push Up – 3 sets of 8

You will need an elevated surface no more than 6" in height. A medicine ball can be used for more difficulty

- o Get into a push up position with both hands on the surface
- o Complete a push up

o Take one hand off of the surface and place it on the floor
o Complete another push up
o Return to the starting position and complete a push up
o Take the other hand off of the surface and place it on the floor
o Complete a push up
o Return to the starting position and complete a push up
o This sequence counts as 1 rep

Fire Hydrant – 3 sets of 15

o Start on your hands and knees
o Keep your hands under your shoulders
o Keep your knees under your hips
o Look directly toward the ground in front of you
o Just as the title says – raise your leg with your knee bent level with your hips
o Complete each group of sets on one leg before switching to the other

**These exercises are to be done Thursday and Saturday
Weeks 2, 4 and 6**

WARM UP – 10 minutes – see the list from Fitness Testing

Power Skip – 5 sets of 3 minutes

- o Raise a knee up toward your hip
- o Reach with opposite hand high over your head
- o Alternate skipping motion with as much power as you can provide
- o Be mindful of uneven surfaces – watch where you are going!

Stairs – 10 sets of 1 minute

- o Climb like there's a million dollars at the top for the first one up the stairs

High Knees – 3 sets of 1 minute

- o Raise your knee just over hip high
- o Lower it
- o Raise the opposite knee just over hip high
- o Lower it
- o Repeat quickly
- o To make this exercise more difficult add a hop between each knee raise and extend the time/sets

Jump Rope – 3 sets of 3 minutes

- o If you do not have a jump rope or just cannot get benefit from this exercise – jump like you have a jump rope
- o To make this exercise more difficult extend your sets and time to 5-7 sets and 5 minute jumping

5 TEN STRETCHES

Stretching is an important part of fitness. Unless you are a high performance athlete ready to engage in the sport of your choice – stretching helps improve your overall fitness levels.

The next 10 common stretches are perfect after a workout. The cool down process is just as important as the workout.

Please remember that if there is any pain – stop!

When you perform your stretches do not bounce. That's old school technique and we prefer to leave that in the past. We have established that the body responds better to a stretch with a hold, not a bounce. Do yourselves a favor and leave the bounce at home!

Hip Flexor Stretch

- o Kneel on the floor and bend both knees.
- o Place your shins on the floor with your foot relaxed behind you.
- o Lunge forward so that your front knee is at a 90° angle
- o Make sure your front knee is directly above your ankle to prevent injury
- o Keep your torso upright and look straight ahead
- o Lean into the stretch.
- o Hold for 30 seconds and gently release
- o Repeat with other side

Seated Twist

- o Sit on the floor
- o Sit up straight. Don't slouch
- o Extend your legs in front of you and lock your knees
- o Keep your ankles and knees together
- o Gently rotate your torso to the right and then the left
- o Repeat 3 sets

Bending Stretch

- o Stand with feet hip width apart
- o Using a sturdy surface to steady yourself on
- o Bend slowly forward from your waist
- o Warp your arms around your legs and hug the
- o Complete for one minute

Butterfly Stretch

- o Sit on floor with your feet together and your knees bent
- o Grab your toes with your hands
- o Slowly lower your body toward your legs
- o Hold this pose for 30 seconds or more

Pigeon on the Ground Stretch

- o Lie on the floor face up
- o Bend your knees
- o Place your feet flat on the floor
- o Cross one leg over the other in an L shape
- o Hood your arms around the leg that has your foot on the floor
- o Gently pull the leg toward your chest
- o Hold this position for 45 seconds or more
- o Gently release
- o Switch legs

Cobra Stretch

- o Lie face down on the ground
- o Place your hands shoulder width apart as if you're going to do a push up
- o Keep your hips on the ground
- o Gently Lift your torso in the air
- o Pull your torso away from the ground gently reaching back
- o Look toward the ceiling
- o Hold this position for 45 seconds or more

Tricep Stretch

- o Extend your arms over your head
- o Bend one elbow
- o Place your palm of that elbow on your neck/upper back

o Reach over the top of your head with the opposite hand grasping just below the elbow
o Gently pull the elbow back toward the back of your head
o Hold this position for 45 seconds or more
o Switch arms

Standing Thigh Stretch

o Stand straight with your feet together
o Steady yourself against a wall or chair if needed
o Bring your heel toward your butt
o Grab the top of your toe with the same side hand
o Gently pull your leg toward your back
o Hold this position for 45 seconds or more
o Switch legs

Prisoner Stretch

o Stand up straight with your feet shoulder width apart
o Place your hands behind your back
o Touch your palms together
o Lock your fingers together
o Gently lean forward while lifting your arms toward the ceiling behind you
o Hold this position for 45 seconds or more

Doorway Stretch

o Stand in a door way with your feet staggered
o One foot in front of the other
o Grasp the door frame on each side with each hand
o Lean toward the front foot until you feel the stretch through your chest and shoulders
o Look up just a touch
o Hold this position for 45 seconds or more
o Switch feet and repeat

Many people fail to place the proper emphasis on stretching. They arrive and do an obligatory warm up and then exercise. That's it. They don't take the time to allow their muscles a chance to cool down.

There is a lot of information out there related to stretching before a workout and it is a question I am asked quite often. My research and belief is that cold stretching – the type of stretching you do when you just show up for your workout, no warm up – just head right into stretching – is not a good idea.

Your muscles need to be warm to gain the length you are typically seeking when you stretch your body. If you wake up, get dressed and drive to the gym only to plop down and engage in five or ten minutes of stretching before you ever do any sort of activity – you're risking injury and probably one of the clients that have constant issues with muscle pulls and strains.

I have a handful of clients that I try to discourage from this activity but they insist. It appears to be more of a social and mental stretch than anything else. They are preparing for the workout and stretching affords them those unjudged moments before they get moving. It would be better to show up and just sit there until you are ready to begin the warm up. However, each person is in charge of their own program. If stretching is what you insist on doing before you warm up your body then hopefully you'll take this opportunity to research and learn more about stretching.

Regardless of your schedule, stretching needs to be included in any workout.

If you are an athlete then you need to do your research. There are several recent studies to suggest that stretching before a big event may actually hinder your performance but again, your body, your decision. Read the studies and do your homework. It may make all of the difference in how your body performs.

Many clients ask me about Yoga. I have tried Yoga and think it has a great deal to offer. Now, don't confuse that with the belief that I participate in the various "wild children" forms of Yoga. I don't. My personal preference is for restorative Yoga. I do enough hardcore physical activity that restorative Yoga affords me the opportunity to go at a slower pace and reap the benefits of calming my system while also challenging it in a more soothing and relaxing way. Check out some Yoga classes. You may like it.

6 FOOD

Food. It is the necessary blissful evil that drives many people to gain a few pounds here and there.

Many people tell me that they LOVE to eat. LOVE food. LOVE everything about it.

I was never that person. I have been working hard at changing my lifelong behavior of devouring my food in a matter of minutes. I like to get it over with and move on. The entire process annoys me. If I were not the type of person that avoids pharmaceuticals – I would prefer a space-age food pill to be taken as needed. Food in general is not a love or passion of mine. Sugar – well that's just an outright addiction so it doesn't count!

As a child I would be the last one allowed to leave the table. MANY nights would be spent staring at a plate of cold food. My family had eaten and gone on to other things while I sat blinking at the detestable mess before me. I hated to eat traditional meals. I was the type of kid that would graze through the day if you let me but when it came time for an actual meal, I dreaded it. I'm not sure if it was the pressure of being one of the last generations that had the expectation of a "clean plate" after a meal or if I didn't like the food or I was just controlling what I felt I could control. I have no idea but what I CAN tell you is that I got into trouble more than once for stuffing my pockets and shoes full of food or pasting various "stickable" foods under the table to avoid having to eat it.

I drove my mother crazy. She always had to fight with me about dinner. I am sure she dreaded it as much as I did but I was stubborn. If I did not want to eat it – I would sit there all night and I recall at least one occasion where I sat from our normal dinner time until my mother was headed off to bed. I refused to eat and by her bedtime, my mother had to give in. My punishment had to be something else because I would have been in the exact same spot until it was time to go to school the next day.

As a small child I tried very hard to be what I was expected to be but in this one area, I couldn't meet the demands. I still can't explain it other than to say I was just not hungry. My father eventually gave up. He insisted that I eat a balanced meal, once I was done he didn't force the issue. It was easier to tell me later when I was hungry that I should have eaten than it was to try to outlast my iron clad anti-food avoidances.

Many children regulate their food needs MUCH better than adults do. As adults we have learned how to override our body's messages. Think about that small child in your family. If they do not want to eat – they will not eat. Plain and simple. Now, that of course is barring any medical issues. The average small child will tell you when they are hungry, thirsty or when they are full. Listen to them and try to learn from them. Our bodies want food when it needs it, fluid when it needs it. Nothing more and nothing less but our minds and emotion decide we need cake or that third bottle of pop.

You need to learn how to reprogram your processes and when you do it, you will find the success that you have been searching for.

Let talk about timing. When should you eat? How much? How often and what types of food should you be consuming regularly?

As you probably know, there is a lot of conflicting information out there regarding our nutritional needs and timing of our meals. Some people thrive with intermittent fasting while others swear by juicing. There are new methods, old methods and the tried and true methods. This book is the latter of the group. I don't embrace the new fads that come and go. If they are not harmful – which many are – then I have no reason to slam those methods. If they are healthy and work, great. If they are unhealthy then they don't really work.

The tried and true method has been around since we decided to become insecure about our shapes and sizes.

It is always going to be basic math. If too much goes in and not enough is expelled – you will gain weight. 2 + 2 will ALWAYS equal 4.

Now, before some of you get riled up – this book is designed with the average person in mind. There are some medical issues that wreak havoc with our bodies and this book is NOT designed to address those issues nor should anyone assume it is.

The average person needs to use simple math to lose weight, gain weight, increase muscle mass, see definition in muscles or any of the other goals one may have.

The majority of people seeking an exercise and diet plan are generally seeking weight loss so we will use this as our focus.

In the next chapter you will be presented with specific meal plans. It is up to you to refine them, discount them or embrace the as they are. You know your body best. Make sure if you are going to substitute, you substitute with an equivalent source and try not to "guesstimate".

This is where a Food Journal comes in handy. You want to record anything and everything you eat or drink on a daily basis. Not only do you want to write down that Cheeseburger but you also want to do the research and write down the calories, fat content, carbohydrates and protein. For some clients with high blood pressure I also have them record salt. Diabetics need to record sugar (MANY people OTHER than diabetics would be advised to also record sugar. You might be stunned when you see the daily totals.)

The percentages that I recommend for my clients are 55% Carbohydrates and then depending on your body's response 20-30% fat and 20-30% protein. If you work out regularly, you need to consider giving your body more protein.

I suggest you shoot for 30-35% of your diet consist of lean protein for fat loss. This applies to those wanting to lose weight or those wanting to retain lean muscle mass. Avoid fatty or fried meats. Those don't count!

Meal prep is the other key to success. In my home I prepare the meal plan on Saturday. We shop and cook on Sunday and prepare the packages for the week. I purchased inexpensive reusable freeze, dishwasher, and microwave safe containers for around $9. They are more along the lines of food service storage containers and work perfectly. You can prepackage your meals, put your date and what the item is on a piece of masking tape and put it in the freezer.

In the morning I remove my lunch meal from the freezer, place it in the refrigerator to thaw. When it's time for lunch I heat it and eat it. Quick, healthy, pre-measured and easy. I have no reason not to eat at home because it is just as fast as any drive-thru and I know my food has wholesome ingredients prepared in sanitary conditions. You can't beat that!

Do your meal prep on your day off and you'll have a worry free week.

Let's take a look at your meal plans!

7 MEAL PLANS AND RECIPES

These meals are for Monday – Wednesday – Friday
Weeks 1, 3 and 5

Meal Prep should be done before the week starts

Breakfast

Old Fashioned Oatmeal with Blueberries & Almonds
¾ cup Old fashioned uncooked oats
1/3 teaspoon honey
¼ cup almond milk or skim milk
¾ tablespoon almonds
½ cup blueberries

Heat the milk and honey to a boil over medium. Stir in oats and allow to cook with occasional stirring for 5 minutes or until oats are thick. Toss in almonds and blueberries when done

Weight loss will not have a snack between Breakfast and Lunch. If you are seeking any other goal you will want to insert a wholesome healthy snack a few hours after breakfast.

Lunch

Avocado Turkey Wrap
1 grain tortilla
½ avocado
5 oz. Turkey breast – deli oven roasted. Try to avoid heavily processed.
Tomato to taste
¼ cup spinach leaves
1 cup raw carrots

Snack
1 Large Apple
2 tablespoons Almond butter

Dinner
(One serving. Multiply measurements by number of servings desired)

Mustard Glazed Chicken
Boneless skinless chicken breast
Light sea salt
Light pepper
Light garlic
½ teaspoon thyme
2 tablespoons Dijon mustard

Place chicken in pan and add seasoning
Spread mustard on chicken
Bake at 400°

Sautéed Mixed vegetables
Can use frozen mix
1 tablespoon olive oil
Dash of sea salt
Sautee vegetables until warm

Seasoning is free. If you want to add something else – do it! Let's keep going.

**These meals are for Tuesday – Thursday - Saturday
Weeks 1, 3 and 5**

Meal Prep should be done before the week starts

Breakfast

Yogurt Parfait

6 oz. Plain Greek Yogurt
1 cup Natures Path Blueberry Flax Cereal
¼ cup blueberries
¼ cup strawberries
1 ½ teaspoon of honey
2 ¾ teaspoon of almonds

Mix ingredients together. Eat cold.

Weight loss will not have a snack between Breakfast and Lunch. If you are seeking any other goal you will want to insert a wholesome healthy snack a few hours after breakfast.

Lunch
Roast Beef Wrap
1 Grain tortilla wrap
5 oz. lean roast beef
½ cup spinach leaves
Tomato to taste
1 thin slice chosen cheese if you wish
1 cup of celery

Snack
1 cup mixed grapes
1 serving of walnuts

Dinner
Salmon and rice
5 oz. salmon
½ teaspoon of olive oil
Add onion to taste or skip if you wish
¼ tablespoon salt
¼ teaspoon oregano
¼ teaspoon rosemary

Heat oven to 450°
Place salmon in pan adding ½ seasoning to top of meat
Bake ½ way through and turn salmon over adding second half of seasoning
Cook until done

1 cup brown rice
Dash of salt

Bring brown rice to boil and allow to cook for about 15 minutes. Remove from heat when done and add dash of salt

If you find you are hungry in the morning between Breakfast and Lunch – try increasing your water intake. Dehydration is a problem with the majority of adults. Research shows that humans struggle with knowing the difference between being hungry and being thirsty.

These meals are for Monday – Wednesday - Friday
Weeks 2, 4 and 6

Meal Prep should be done before the week starts

Breakfast

Cereal & Eggs
Cereal:
½ cup Natures Path Blueberries Flax Cereal
½ cup Skim Milk
½ cup Blueberries

Eggs:
3 egg whites
¾ tablespoon of chosen cheese

Weight loss will not have a snack between Breakfast and Lunch. If you are seeking any other goal you will want to insert a wholesome healthy snack a few hours after breakfast.

Lunch
Salmon salad
5 oz. grilled salmon
3 cups mixed spring salad
Tomato to taste
2 tablespoon almonds
2/3 cup mixed grapes
½ cup cucumber
½ cup zucchini
2 tablespoons vinaigrette

Snack

Pear
1 cup cottage cheese

Dinner
Grilled steak
¼ pound sirloin steak
Dash of pepper
1 teaspoon garlic powder
1 teaspoon thyme
1 teaspoon all spice

Add all ingredients in a small bowl. Toss a handful of ingredients on the bottom of a pan. Place steak in pan and empty the rest of the spices on the steak. Broil until done.

Sautéed nutty broccoli

1 ½ cup fresh broccoli
1 tablespoon pine nuts (can sub walnuts or almonds)
1 teaspoon olive oil
Dash of salt

Combine ingredients in pan over medium heat. Stir occasionally and remove when broccoli is tender. Average is 6 minutes

By now you should be adapting to the meal plans. If you notice, there are not calories or numbers to reference. I have left these out so that you are forced to review, research and record this information on your own. By repetitive actions we begin to reestablish what a proper serving is and become knowledgeable about what nutrition components our food contains.

**These meals are for Monday – Wednesday - Friday
Weeks 2, 4 and 6**

Meal Prep should be done before the week starts

Breakfast
Waffles and Almonds with Berries on top

1 whole grain waffle

6 oz. Greek plain yogurt

3 tablespoons Almonds

¾ cup blueberries

1 tablespoon honey

Weight loss will not have a snack between Breakfast and Lunch. If you are seeking any other goal you will want to insert a wholesome healthy snack a few hours after breakfast.

Lunch

Turkey Sandwich

2 slices grain bread

5 oz. turkey breast – avoid processed if possible

½ cup spinach leaves

1 teaspoon mustard

1 thin slice chosen cheese if you wish

Snacks

1 Tablespoon Almond butter

1 Graham Cracker sheet

Dinner

Broiled Scallops
4 oz. scallops
½ tablespoon honey
Dash of salt
¼ teaspoon garlic powder
½ teaspoon lemon juice
½ teaspoon lime juice

Combine seasoning and juice in a bowl. Clean and dry scallops and add to mix. Allow to sit 24 hours if possible making sure to mix the bowl every so often.

Broil scallops until opaque throughout and lightly browned

Sautéed spinach
6 oz. spinach leaves
½ teaspoon garlic
Dash of sea salt
½ teaspoon of olive oil

Combine all ingredients in the pan and heat until spinach is just wilted and serve right away.
1 small baked sweet potato

Notes:

8 FORMS

Now that you have reviewed the book and know what is happening it is time for the hard part. You need to keep track of what you are doing in order to meet your goals. Food and exercise journals are the best way to own your progress.

Sure you can download an app and sometime soon I may offer one as well but part of my resistance to going digital has been that there is a disconnect from what you eat and what you know about it. Researching and writing down your food and activity seems to have a much large impact on a client than scanning something in and seeing the numbers registered on a screen. The true connection isn't there.

That is why there are journal examples in this book. I want you to write down what you eat and the activities that you do. I want you to research how many calories you burned on a 2 mile walk or how many you consumed when you ate a candy bar.

Get a journal and start recording right away.

We will start with the food journal. Exercise is has extreme value in your fitness level and longevity but nutrition is where the battle is won.

Look at it this way – and I have said this countless times.

If you put watered down stale bad gas in your cars tank, your car will not run well.

Your body is not a lot different. Good nutrition yields the results you want.

Having said that, no one expects you to be 100% perfect. You will have days where your plan is the last thing you want to follow. Cravings will nag at you. (Hint: Cravings last 10-20 minutes on average. Drink some water and engage in another activity. Get busy and the craving will go away.) If you give in to cravings, it is normal. Just try to manage them because as you make allowance after allowance you end up derailing your program.

Look at it this way – and yes, I have said this countless times before;

If you are driving and get a flat tire will you won't stop the car and flatten the other tires. You'll fix it and move on.

Cravings are the same thing. If you decide to have that donut it doesn't mean you need to throw in the towel for the entire day. It's a donut. It isn't arsenic. Well, nutritionists would disagree but – you know what I mean.

You have to allow yourself the chance to fail in order to have the chance to succeed. The majority of people will struggle with food choices. Many of those choices are based on emotions.

Start recognizing what motivates a craving or "the hell with it" attitude that everyone faces at some point. If you can recognize your triggers then you can work to find an alternative or eliminate that coping method.

To do your journal you will need to know the math. Don't worry, it's pretty basic and there is an example on the sheet.

Each gram of fat is 9 calories. Each gram of protein and carbs are 4 calories. Take your grams and multiply it by the proper number. This gives you your calories. Divide each of those numbers into your total calories and you will have your percentages. Please don't fret if you don't get 100%. That's normal.

In order to be successful you have to own your behaviors. You have to own your commitment and you have to own your follow through.

Here are the tools you need for each of those!

The Fat Trainer® Food Journal

Date	Food	Calories	Fat(g)	Carb(g)	Protein(g)
12/25	8 oz. Turkey	305	1.6	0	67.9
12/25	4 oz. baby carrots	40	.2	9.3	.7
12/25	1oz cheddar cheese	69	5.6	.2	4.2
				Grams X 9	Grams X 4	Grams X 4
		Calories	Fat	Carbs	Protein
		414	7.4	9.5	72.8
	Total Calories		66.7	38	292.2
	Total %	414	16%	9%	71%

The Fat Trainer® Food Journal

Date	Food	Calories	Fat(g)	Carb(g)	Protein(g)
		Calories	Fat	Carbs	Protein
	Total Calories				
	Total %				

The Fat Trainer® Exercise Journal

Date	Exercise	Time	Weight	Sets	Reps	Calories
12/25	Bike	90min	–	–	–	745
12/26	Bench Pr	–	113	3	12	NA
						Calories
	Totals					745

The Fat Trainer® Exercise Journal

Date	Exercise	Time	Weight	Sets	Reps	Calories
						Calories
	Totals					

9 KNOWLEDGE

You have your tools, you have the meal plan, the exercise plan.

How do you make it all work?

You stick to the meal plan
You stick to the exercise plan
You write down what you eat or drink
You write down when you exercise

Each and every one of these are a key to your success. To make them work you need to use them.

Each day off you want to complete your meal prep for the week. Not planning ahead is one of the biggest reasons for failure I hear.

Package your food for work or road trips. Keep your journal with you through the day. Remember why you are doing what you are doing and your goals will be met.

Tip 1
Go grocery shopping for your plan

Don't forget containers to keep your meals in. Reusable are best.

Tip 2
Do your meal prep no matter what. That way you can grab your food on the go and stay on track. Failure to make yourself do food prep will likely result in being crunched for time and allow poor food choices to be made.

Tip 3
If you are someone who never works out after a work, do it first thing in the morning. Getting your workout done is a sense of accomplishment and often yields better decisions through the day. You don't want that set of stairs to be for nothing by eating that package of cookies!

Tip 4
Keep track of your water consumption. Water is key for life. You won't live long without it and your body needs it to lose weight. More on that shortly.

Tip 5

Write your food and exercise activity down in your journal. Your starting points are fantastic motivators when you are feeling down or the scale isn't budging like you think it should.

Tip 6

Write your totals in your food journal as you go. Don't wait until the end of the day to see where your numbers fall. You need to be proactive. Being aware of your numbers as you go will make a world of difference.

Tip 7

Get a water app or line up water on your desk to remind you to drink. As I mentioned, water is a key source when it comes to life and weight loss. If you are like me and struggle with consuming enough water, making it visible or having an app that pesters you helps your consumption and obtaining your goals.

Tip 8

Without sleep you will struggle with your goals. Our bodies need sleep. Failure to provide enough restorative sleep has been shown to cause weight gain. Do your research. Get some Z's and you'll find that staying on track is much easier.

Tip 9

If you have sugar craving that is driving you up a wall try to drink water and distract yourself for 10-20 minutes. The cravings usually go away. Repeat to yourself "I want to hit my goals. It's just a candy bar. I don't NEED it, I want it and it won't help me reach my goals."

Tip 10

Stress weighs you down. Literally. Like sleep, too much stress has been shown to cause weight gain. There is tons of research on the topic and as you know, stress can damage your body. Practice self-care techniques. One of the most natural stress relievers is – exercise. It's true! Look it up!

10 PARTING WORDS

No one wants to fail and really, you don't have to. Tell as many people as you can that you are starting a new program (and feel free to share where they can get their copy!) and ask them to help hold you accountable.

Enlisting your friends, co-workers and family will help you succeed and likely cause others within your circle to begin the process of transformation.

Motivation is also a key element. Find what motivates you. Is it getting into a smaller size before spring? Gaining muscle mass before summer? Whatever it is you need to write it on a note and place that note where you will see it the most. For many of us that is our desk at work. You will see it every day and during key times you will focus on it and that is important. Being motivated makes all of the difference in anything in life and for a transformation – it is crucial.

Listen, I know it isn't easy. I've been where you are. I have my own trials and tribulations that I have to deal with – just like you. I get busy and don't do my meal prep and then I spend the week regretting it and trying to play catch up. I hate that! So then I carve out time on my day off to make sure I get it done because it makes my life so much easier.

Exercise isn't always fun but it is necessary. Refining your diet is even more so. The old saying that the gym is 10% because the other 90% is the kitchen is true. A crappy diet yields crappy results. So clean up your diet and stay focused.

Gain an insight into why you "fall off the wagon". Is it because you are angry? Because you are bored or socially – that's what you do? By learning more about what drives you to overindulge you'll be able to take the steps to find a way to cope better and also be able to recognize what is truly happening.

No one wants to feel like they are the biggest or most out of shape person in a room. You can use this plan to change your body but also your self-image. It's pretty exciting when you think about it!

My suggestions are that you write down your beginning stats, take a beginning picture, write down your measurements and keep track. Every month you should retest your fitness level, record your stats/measurements and take another picture. Those things will be a cherished possession when you get to the end of your road and look back. It is also valuable for the times you are discouraged and want to quit. You're able to take out your starting information and see how much progress you've made. That has saved more than one client on more than one occasion. I think you'll find it valuable too.

You may find The Fat Trainer® Exercise Journal useful. It's available!
Keep your eye out for Volume 2 of The Fat Trainer ® Plan and our app due out next year.

YOU decide if you are ready. YOU decide if you can do this or not and if you were not sure – you wouldn't have bought the book!

Stick to your plan. Stick to your goals. You can do this!

Notes:

Journal

Journal

Journal

Journal

Journal

Journal

Journal

Journal

Journal

Journal

Journal

Journal

Journal

Journal

Journal

Journal

Journal

Journal

Journal

Journal

Journal

Journal

Journal

Journal

Journal

Journal

Journal

ABOUT THE AUTHOR

Laura was close to 270 pounds when she made the decision to lose weight. She took control of her situation and spent a great deal of time becoming educated in fitness training. Laura is a NASM Certified Personal Trainer with experience in boot camps, personal training, general group training, general nutrition, senior fitness with her current specialty in weight loss.

In her free time Laura enjoys many different activities and believes a wide variety of interests keeps you focused on fitness. "I couldn't just run on a treadmill day after day. It's great for those that can but I must have exercise A.D.D., I need to be doing something different to stay engaged. I try to incorporate that into my training programs for clients."

Laura has won national and local awards for excellence and her commitment to fitness and says that her greatest accomplishment is each and every time a client has reached a goal or accomplished something they never thought possible. "I love seeing my clients try new things that they swore they could never do only to find out that they do the activity but did it very well. That is the best part of what I do!"

Watch for more books from Laura in the future. She has a Volume 2 for her The Fat Trainer® Diet and Exercise series in the works as well as an app due next year.

Change happens over time

Give yourself the gift of patience

Laura

www.ingramcontent.com/pod-product-compliance
Lightning Source LLC
Chambersburg PA
CBHW060634290526
45793CB00001B/241